Preface

The right to abortion is under concerted attack. The White House, Congress, state legislatures, and the courts have all joined in the bipartisan attempt to curtail the right of women to control their own bodies. Catholic bishops and Protestant fundamentalist preachers have helped lead the charge. This has put wind in the sails of right-wing foes of abortion, who have bombed dozens of abortion clinics and regularly harass and intimidate women seeking abortions.

To justify these reactionary moves, and to prepare the way for further blows to the constitutional right to abortion, a propaganda campaign has been unleashed in the big-business media to brand abortion as murder, and women who have abortions as murderers. The purpose of this campaign is to erode majority support for legal abortion as the cutting edge of a broader assault on women's struggle for equality.

Now, more than ever, supporters of women's equality need to counter these reactionary ideas with a clear defense of abortion rights and an explanation of the stake that women and working people have in the fight to keep abortion safe, legal, and available.

This pamphlet is intended to be part of the effort to defend abortion rights. It is designed to be circulated broadly—on the job, among unionists, Blacks, Latinos, family farmers, and students. It answers the antiabortion propaganda of the ruling class and provides a basic explanation of why working people should support abortion rights. It is also intended for use by women's rights activists, who will find it a valuable source of information and political argumentation in the fight to defend abortion rights.

Pat Grogan
July 1985

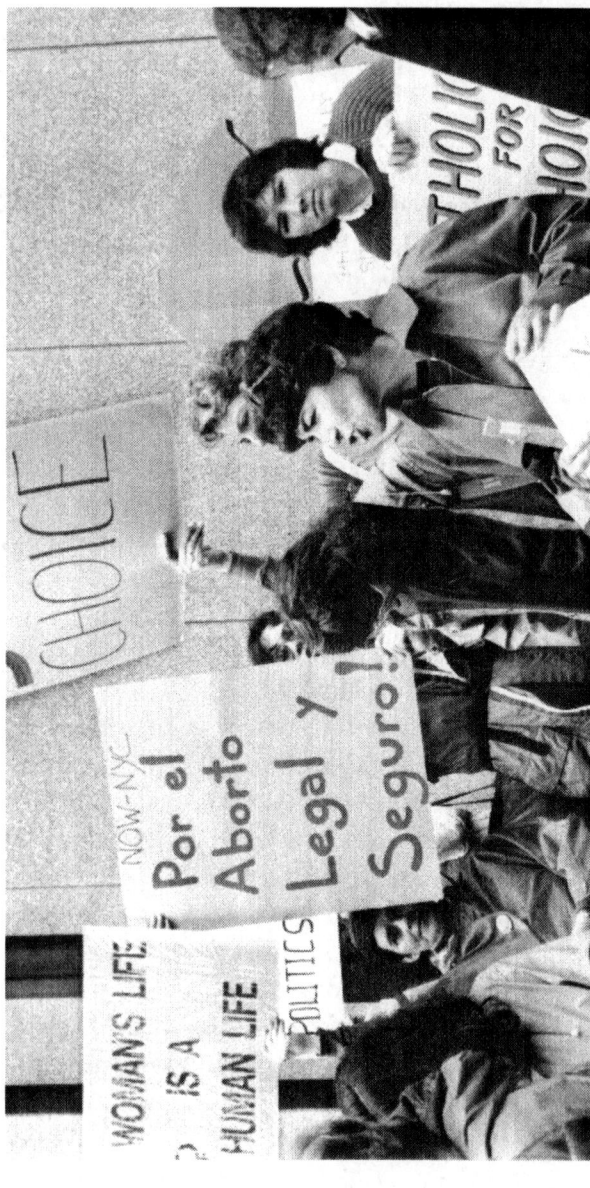

June 8, 1985, march to St. Patrick's Cathedral in New York City for abortion rights, organized by the National Organization for Women.

The issue is women's rights

BY PAT GROGAN

On January 22, 1973, women won their most important victory in decades.

The U.S. Supreme Court, in *Roe vs. Wade,* ruled that women had the constitutional right to have abortions. The ruling legalized abortion through the first twenty-four weeks of pregnancy and struck down all laws that restricted that right.

For the first time the right of *women* to decide whether or not to bear children—not the state, church, husband, father, or priest—was recognized.

The women's liberation movement saw reproductive freedom as the most fundamental right of women, a precondition for full equality and liberation. Without the right to control her own body, a woman could not exercise effective control over her life.

Beginning in the 1960s, contraception was becoming more available and accepted, but it was not foolproof—and still isn't. Advances in medical science had made abortion a safe, simple, medical procedure. But in most states, abortion was against the law. Women were forced to bear children against their will, or risk dangerous—and often deadly—illegal or self-induced abortions.

In 1969, the year before New York State adopted liberalized abortion laws—a step that laid the basis for the later Supreme Court victory—approximately *210,000* women entered city hospitals due to abortion complications.

The restrictions on abortion were powerful and barbaric chains on women. Black women and Latinas suffered the most from the illegal status of abortion. *Eighty percent* of the hundreds of women who died each year were Black and Spanish-speaking women.

And many Black women and Latinas were forced to submit to sterilization in order to obtain an abortion.

Prior to the emergence of the feminist movement in the late 1960s, many supporters of legal abortion presented their arguments in terms of population control—arguments that are used to bolster the racist practice of forced sterilization.

The feminist movement put the axis for the fight to legalize abortion where it belonged—on the right of women to control their own bodies. It was on this basis that majority support for legal abortion was won.

Because of the stakes involved in the fight for abortion rights, this right was never secure.

Several years ago, Democrats and Republicans alike began to step up their attacks on the right to abortion.

The Hyde Amendment, passed by Congress in 1976, was the most serious blow. It cut off Medicaid funding for abortions, except in cases of rape, incest, or when a woman's life is in danger. In May 1981, Congress cut off funds even in cases of rape and incest.

In October 1984, Congress once again denied abortion funding for victims of rape and incest.

Since the Hyde Amendment was passed, thirty-six states have cut off state funding for abortions.

This strikes hardest at Black women, Latinas, and the poorest women. It is part of the attack against the right of all women to abortion and lays the basis for further attempts to restrict abortion rights.

In the years 1978 and 1979 alone, almost 1.5 million women were unable to obtain abortions, either because of lack of facilities or inability to pay.

These attacks against women's rights have sharply escalated in the last few years.

There were 180 incidents of violent attacks by right-wing foes of abortion rights on abortion clinics as of November 1984. This includes 20 arsons and firebombings.

Women seeking abortions are harassed, threatened, and called "murderers" by "right-to-lifers" who try to create an atmosphere of fear and intimidation at abortion clinics. They are the shock troops of a broader assault on abortion rights.

The 1984 presidential elections were used as a staging ground for a major escalation in the ideological offensive against women's rights. The main theme sounded was, "Abortion is murder!"

The Catholic archbishops pressed to make abortion the "key issue" in the elections. Fundamentalist Protestant preachers like "Moral Majority" leader Jerry Falwell stepped up their antiabortion propaganda.

Reagan and the Republican Party convention openly endorsed legislation that would "make clear that the 14th Amendment protections apply to unborn children."

Prominent liberal Democrats like Geraldine Ferraro responded by agreeing that abortion is murder, but that as long as a majority supports abortion rights, it shouldn't be made illegal.

"I do not believe in abortion," Ferraro emphatically told the press. "I am opposed to abortion as a Catholic . . . but I will not impose my religious views on others."

The question, however, is not separation of church and state. The question is a woman's right to abortion.

Throughout the campaign, Ferraro stressed her abhorrence of abortion, helping to strengthen the reactionary "abortion is murder" campaign against women.

Week after week, abortion is discussed in the big-business media as a moral, religious, ethical, and scientific question; a private, public, personal, and medical question. But the real issue is the right of women to decide if and when to have children.

The torrent of antiabortion propaganda does not come out of a big victory by the capitalist rulers against women's rights. Rather it is aimed at launching a fight to reverse the gains women have won in the last 15 years.

The steps taken toward equality by both the women's rights movement and the civil rights movement have strengthened the entire working class in its ability to struggle against the employers.

In order to lay the basis for ever deeper attacks against the rights and living standards of the working class—and as part of the preparation for full-scale imperialist war in Central America—the ruling class must pit worker against worker, using racist and sexist prejudices to undermine the unity and strength of the working class.

The ruling class ideological offensive is aimed at undermining the powerful idea that *women should have equal rights.* It is aimed at convincing both men and women that a woman's place is in the home, and that the family, not the government, should bear the cost of caring for children, the sick, and the elderly.

It is aimed at justifying lower pay for women who work and making unemployment of women more acceptable.

The fire is aimed particularly at abortion rights because the right of women to choose whether or not to bear children is an elementary precondition for women's liberation.

Leading the pack of the opponents of abortion rights has been New York's Cardinal John O'Connor.

In a major speech delivered on October 15, 1984, entitled "Human Lives, Human Rights," O'Connor laid out many of the arguments in the antiabortion, anti-women's rights arsenal. These arguments need to be rebutted—forcefully and publicly— by supporters of women's rights.

The theme of O'Connor's speech was the argument that abortion is a social *evil* and that fighting against abortion rights is progressive—like fighting against racism or for the rights of the elderly.

"No one in public life," said O'Connor, "would admit to being a racist or a warmonger." How then, he asks, can anyone justify "putting babies to death?"

O'Connor put an equal sign between abortion and his list of social ills: homelessness, mistreatment of the elderly, drug abuse, pornography, sexual exploitation, child abuse, racism, and war.

By linking abortion to genuine social wrongs and injustices, O'Connor tries to make his reactionary campaign against women's rights more acceptable to the millions of working people who, in their majority, support legal abortion. He tries to paint it up as a new "civil rights" movement.

But abortion is not an injustice—it is a basic human right. The right of women to control their own bodies—which is what is at stake in the fight over legal abortion—is an elementary precondition for the liberation of women from the oppression they suffer as a sex.

It is the women's liberation movement, which championed the fight for abortion rights, that is kindred to the fight for civil rights and against Washington's war.

Women's liberation and civil rights fighters stand together against inequality, discrimination, and exploitation. Both immeasurably strengthen the capacity of the labor movement to resist the current employer-class offensive.

O'Connor bases his arguments on the charge that abortion is murder and that women who have abortions are, therefore, guilty of murdering children.

Abortion is not murder. It is a simple medical procedure that terminates a pregnancy. Abortion is key to allowing women to decide whether and when to bear children.

One of the hierarchy's favorite arguments is to liken what O'Connor calls the "murder" of "one and a half million unborn human lives . . . every year" to Hitler's Holocaust—the Nazi policy of mass murder of Jews and others. He does not mention that as part of the Nazis' degradation of human life, they outlawed abortion and contraception, reducing women to the status of breeders whose role was bearing children, and whose only place was in the kitchen and in church.

By saying the issue is the "rights" of the unborn, O'Connor and Company try to sucker people into a pointless, hairsplitting argument about the exact moment when human life begins. This is a total diversion from the real issue: the right of women to control their own bodies.

O'Connor's pose as a champion of "human lives, human rights" does not include a concern for the lives and rights of women.

With a wave of the hand, he dismisses as untrue the "impression" that "masses" of women would die if abortion were to be made illegal again.

"We are informed," he blithely asserts, "that this is not supported by figures issued by the United States government."

This is a lie. Official statistics show that during the 1960s, when abortion was illegal, *thousands* of women were maimed and *hundreds* died each year as a result of botched abortions. We have no way of knowing how many other abortion mortalities were reported as deaths due to "severe hemorrhaging" or "miscarriage."

In fact, it was outrage at the killings and maimings resulting from illegal abortion that helped spur women to demand an end to antiabortion laws. Legal abortions save lives—women's lives.

O'Connor's denigration of the value of women's lives comes through clearly when he discusses why a woman should be forced to bear a child, no matter what the circumstances under which she becomes pregnant.

"Certainly rape," he concedes, "is always a frightening possibility." But, he asks, "Is it at least *possible* that bearing a child, however conceived . . . might bring, even out of the tragedy of rape, a rich fulfillment?"

Forcing a woman to bear a child against her will is a brutal denial of a woman's humanity and dignity.

Bearing a child affects all the other aspects and decisions of a woman's life—her ability to get an education, get a better job—or any job. As long as women are vulnerable to unwanted pregnancies, breaking down economic and social barriers on the job, in education, and in the home becomes a much more difficult task.

Of course, legalized abortion cannot solve all the problems facing women. But the right to choose is the most fundamental step toward women being able to achieve full equality.

That's why after women began pouring into the work force in the last three decades, the question of legalizing abortion became a burning issue for millions. When women can control their childbearing functions, it allows them to begin to participate more fully in all aspects of social life. The right to choose means qualitatively more freedom and mobility for women.

We've already seen this in the 12 years that abortion has been legal. Even though access to it is far from universal, it has meant significant changes in the lives of millions of women.

This change in the scope of women's choices led to demands for even greater freedom and opportunity, to a fight for full control by women over their minds and lives as well as their bodies. Encouraged by the abortion-rights victory in 1973, women stepped up their fight for child care, affirmative action, the Equal Rights Amendment, equal pay, and other rights.

O'Connor knows this. In fact, the reason he is so vehemently opposed to abortion rights is precisely because it does challenge the key idea used to justify women's inequality—women's ability to bear children means they are inherently inferior. As a mouthpiece for the ruling class, O'Connor wants to help "keep women in their place" and discourage them—and others—from fighting for their rights.

Not content with labeling women as murderers of the unborn, O'Connor goes one step further.

"We are already seeing cruel signs of what an abortion mentality can mean for all society," he warns. "Again we ask, how safe will the retarded be, the handicapped, the aged, the wheelchaired, the incurably ill, when the so-called 'quality of life' becomes the determinant of who is to live and who is to die?"

This theme is echoed by others, among them Nat Hentoff, a writer for the liberal New York weekly, the *Village Voice*. In an October 2, 1984, article attacking abortion, Hentoff refers to the fetus as the "kid down there."

Hentoff claims that for some women, "because the kid down there is going to be retarded," or "the kid has some other defect," that "the kid is done away with."

Hentoff—like the archbishop—explains that it is a short step from "killing the 'kid down there' to killing an imperfect child that has already been born, or doing away with the handicapped, or the mentally ill, or the retarded."

This absurd slander turns reality on its head.

Since abortion was legalized, there has been no mass slaughter of the sick, aged, or the mentally ill by women.

And the right of a woman to safe, legal abortion has *nothing* to do with euthanasia or treatment of the handicapped.

Far from denigrating the value of human life, treating women as human beings by giving them control over their own bodies enhances the value placed on human life.

O'Connor and Hentoff both try to trivialize the right to abortion by saying women have abortions because having children would be "inconvenient."

Most women, Hentoff says, do not get abortions because they are too poor or young to raise children. This, he believes, while not justifying abortion, would at least explain why a woman would have one.

But, says Hentoff, "For some it is just plain inconvenient, at a particular time in their lives, to have a baby."

The *Village Voice* printed a page full of letters by angry women responding to Hentoff.

"What right has Hentoff to caricature and trivialize the motives of women like this? Is an unwanted child merely an 'inconvenience,' nothing more devastating? Is there no . . . pain worth mentioning in bearing a retarded child?" wrote one reader.

Underlying Hentoff's and O'Connor's view of abortion rights is the assumption that a woman's primary role is in the home, bearing and raising children. Women's desire for personal liberty is reduced to a matter of "convenience" by the likes of Hentoff and O'Connor.

O'Connor especially pounds away at the theme that abortion is racist. "Why have laws against racism when . . . liberal abortion policies amount to another form of subjugation of poor black people?" he asks.

This is false.

As with every aspect of the oppression of women, Black women and Latinas suffer the most from laws restricting the right or access to abortion.

Eighty percent of the women who died at the hands of back-alley abortionists were Black and Spanish-speaking women.

It is Black women and Latinas who suffer the most from laws restricting government funding for abortions.

O'Connor puts an equal sign between the slave laws that oppressed millions of Blacks and the legalization of abortion, which freed millions of women from unwanted pregnancies.

Under slavery, Black women were forced to bear children against their will and were used as breeders to enrich the plantation owners. Black women have been fighting for centuries for the right to control their own bodies. The fight against forced sterilization is the other side of the coin in this struggle. Forced sterilization is the racist practice of coercing women into having an irreversible operation that prevents them from ever getting pregnant again.

It was women's rights fighters, basing themselves firmly on the right of women to control their own bodies, who joined civil rights activists in exposing and combating forced sterilization.

The women's liberation movement rejected the racist "population control" schemes that were used to justify forced sterilization. Laws making abortion illegal and laws that restrict access of poor women to abortion make it easier for racist doctors to demand sterilization as the price for an abortion.

Black women and Latinas have the most to gain from the fight for women's rights because they suffer the double edge of both racist and sexist oppression. That's why a majority of Blacks support legal abortion.

O'Connor also argues against those who say that passing laws against abortion is not an effective way to stop abortion, because women will continue to have them whether or not it is legal.

"It is obvious," O'Connor says, "that law is not the entire answer to abortion. Nor is it the answer to theft, arson, child abuse, or shooting police officers. Everybody knows that. But who would suggest that we repeal laws against such crimes because the laws are so often broken?"

"Is it outlandish to think," he asks, "that laws against abortions might have *some* protective effect?"

O'Connor is right about one thing.

Laws against abortion won't stop women from getting abortions. But laws making abortion illegal will stop *some* women. And they will stop women from getting *safe* abortions.

Women have had and will continue to have abortions to end unwanted pregnancies. The question is whether they will be open, legal, and safe—or secret, illegal, physically dangerous, and psychologically destructive?

O'Connor and the entire hierarchy of the Catholic Church play on people's religious beliefs in an attempt to enlist them in the reactionary campaign against abortion rights and women's equality. They cloak themselves in a phony concern for the poor, the oppressed, and the downtrodden, while they work with all their might to keep the oppressed and exploited on their knees.

All working people have a big stake in answering these attacks on abortion rights.

Interview with Canada's Dr. Henry Morgentaler

BY PAT GROGAN

A determined fight for abortion rights is being waged in both English Canada and the oppressed French-speaking nation of Quebec. Fighters for women's rights in the United States, who are facing relentless attacks against the right to abortion here, can learn important lessons and draw strength from the battle being waged in Canada.

Those forces that have been working to deny women the right to safe, legal abortion in Canada—the federal government; the governments of several of Canada's 10 provinces; the courts; the police; the Catholic Church hierarchy; and the right-wing, "right to life" organizations—are encountering deep resistance.

In both English Canada and Quebec, women's rights fighters, unionists, students, and others are fighting back—including by organizing the largest demonstrations for abortion rights in Canada's history. New abortion rights coalitions have been organized in many cities, and Canada's labor movement has joined the struggle in an active way.

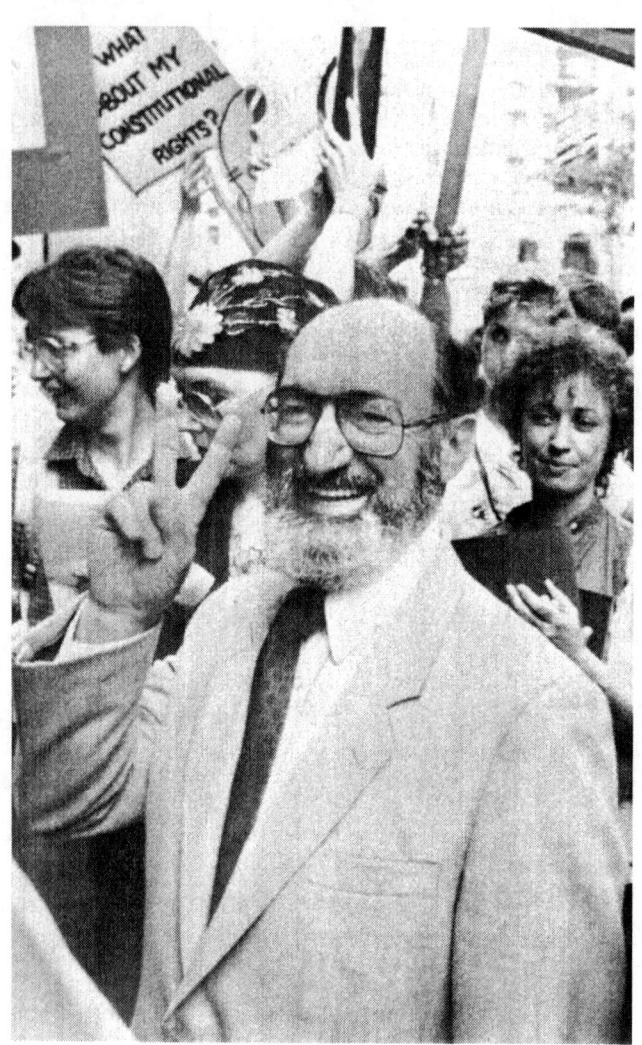

Dr. Henry Morgentaler

Not only have supporters of abortion rights organized to meet new attacks, they have taken the offensive. A renewed campaign to defy and challenge Canada's highly restrictive federal abortion law has gained steam. This struggle takes the form of a fight to establish and maintain abortion clinics separate from hospitals, which are illegal under present law.

In 1969, Canada's laws were changed to make abortion legal, but only under very restricted conditions.

Under the Criminal Code, abortions are only legal if performed in hospitals that have been specially accredited to perform them through the establishment of a Therapeutic Abortion Committee (TAC). Such committees are not mandatory, however, and only one-third of Canada's hospitals have set up TACs, thus permitting them to provide abortions.

The law does not recognize the right of a woman to choose abortion. To get an abortion, a woman must get the consent of the TAC, which is composed of three physicians. Under the law, an abortion may only be granted if the continuation of the pregnancy is considered dangerous to the life and health of the woman.

This law severely restricts access to abortion. In 1983, for example, an estimated 20 percent of the hospitals that do have TACs refused to authorize or perform a single abortion. Access varies widely throughout the country, and in some areas legal abortion is completely unavailable.

Women are subjected to the arbitrary decisions of the TACs, whose members may or may not choose to grant an abortion. Many hospitals limit the number of abortions they will perform. Delays of six to eight weeks are common, forcing women to undergo an abortion later in the pregnancy, when the procedure becomes more complicated and potentially dangerous.

Dr. Henry Morgentaler, a Montreal physician, has been a key figure in the long struggle to break the shackles of this law.

Morgentaler is a survivor of the Nazi concentration camps of Dachau and Auschwitz. He emigrated to Canada in the 1950s.

In 1973 Morgentaler first defied the restrictive law by publicly declaring that he had performed abortions outside a hospital, without the approval of any committee. He argued that abortion is a woman's right.

Three times the government of Quebec Province brought him to trial, and three times Quebec juries refused to convict him. Despite this he spent ten months in jail, where he suffered a heart attack after being beaten by a prison guard and thrown into the "hole."

Finally in 1976, the Parti Quebecois (PQ)—which held a position favoring independence for Quebec—was elected to office on the crest of militant struggles by the Quebecois people. It declared that there would henceforth be no prosecutions of doctors who provide abortions. Since that time, women in Quebec have been able to obtain abortions on demand in clinics and health centers, and government-funded abortions are performed in hospitals, although this is formally a violation of the law.

Canada has a parliamentary system of government. The two major capitalist parties are the Liberals and the Conservatives (commonly known as Tories). The New Democratic Party (NDP) is Canada's Labor Party, based on the unions. Nine of Canada's ten provinces—including Quebec—have governments run by capitalist parties. The exception is the province of Manitoba, where an NDP government was elected. Under the Canadian system, the federal criminal code is administered by each of the provincial governments, and the attorney general of each province has the right to decide whether or not to enforce a federal law, and may decide not to prosecute, as was done in Quebec.

In 1983 Morgentaler announced a new challenge to the federal law and opened two clinics outside of Quebec: one in Toronto, Ontario, and the other in Winnipeg, Manitoba. He was brought to trial in Toronto, and for the fourth time a Canadian jury acquitted him. At present the not-guilty verdict is being appealed by the Ontario government.

In Manitoba, the NDP government—despite the fact that the NDP has a strong, official position favoring abortion rights—has recently waged a vicious campaign against the clinic, twice raiding it and stealing the equipment, and slapping Morgentaler with an injunction preventing him from practicing medicine in the province. This has prevented the clinic from operating.

The fight to establish the clinics in English Canada, protect the gains in Quebec, and bring down the federal law is growing.

Women's rights groups are more and more being joined by unions—from steelworkers to auto workers to public service workers—that are being actively drawn into the battle. The 800,000-strong Ontario Federation of Labor (the equivalent of a state affiliate of the AFL-CIO), reflecting the strong sentiment for women's rights among the ranks of labor, has become involved in the struggle. At the summer 1984 convention of the New Democratic Party, it was the unions and the women's committees that led a successful struggle to win the NDP to the fight to defend the Ontario clinic.

In Quebec, also, the strong pro-women's rights, prochoice positions of the unions are beginning to be tapped. There is a growing consciousness in Quebec that the gains made there are not secure as long as the federal law stands, and that a united movement for abortion rights across Canada is needed. Students in Quebec are taking the lead in organizing to defend the gains in Quebec, and reach out to working people in English Canada.

Representatives from abortion-rights and women's rights organizations from both English Canada and Quebec have mapped out a fight to bring down the restrictive law and win abortion rights.

The following interview with Dr. Morgentaler was obtained on April 2, 1985, on a flight from Toronto to Montreal. In the few hours I spent with Dr. Morgentaler in the airports and on the plane, no less than ten people came over to wish him well, give encouragement, and ask how things were going. Others smiled and waved. As we were leaving the plane, a flight attendant said, "Au revoir, on vous supporte" (Good-bye, we support you).

* * *

MILITANT: You have been involved in the struggle for abortion rights for almost two decades. Can you describe how you became involved?

DR. HENRY MORGENTALER: I started doing general practice in Montreal in 1955, and as a doctor doing replacement work on weekends and nights, I was called to emergencies. One night I had a twenty-two-year-old girl at three o'clock in the morning who had had a bad abortion. She was white as a sheet, she had no blood pressure, she was barely conscious, and from the story I got, she had had an abortion by some incompetent non-doctor. It was clear that she would die if I didn't hospitalize her.

This was not an uncommon occurrence in the fifties. Whole wards of hospitals were filled with women who had either self-induced abortions, or had gone to whoever would offer them that help. It was a major health hazard. About fifteen years ago, the World Health Organization estimated that every year 100,000 women were dying around the world as a result of botched or self-induced abortions. A real epidemic.

And when I talked to my colleagues, they would say, "Well, you know Henry, there's not much you can do about that. If you ever did, you'd be struck from the register, you'd go to jail." The penalty for helping a woman with an unwanted pregnancy was life imprisonment. It is still the same today.

MILITANT: What was the first step you took to change the situation?

MORGENTALER: In 1967 I presented a brief in the name of three humanist groups to the House of Commons Health Committee, which was debating about changing the abortion laws in Canada. And for the first time in a public body, I declared that the right to a safe, medical abortion should be granted to women as a *right,* not a privilege.

What happened then, I didn't predict, but should have. As a result of the publicity that surrounded my appearing on radio, TV, and panels, people came to know my opinions on the subject and women would look me up in the yellow pages, where I was listed as a doctor. And women started coming to my office and would say, "Doctor, I know you are sympathetic. I am pregnant, I can't possibly go through with this pregnancy. Will you help me?"

And I would say, "Yes, it's true I sympathize with you, but I can't help you. I might have to go to jail, it's a crime. It took me a long time to get my medical license. I'm married, I have two children. I'm sorry, I can't help you."

And these women would go out feeling sad, but understanding. And so this parade of women was coming through my office all the time for a number of months, and I started feeling like a coward and a hypocrite. I had a very big struggle with my conscience. And from time to time there were newspaper stories that were terrible. I remember one that said a young woman got pregnant by her boyfriend and asked him to abort her. And since she didn't know how, she encouraged him to use a bicycle pump to push air into the uterus. And she died on the spot, from air embolism. And the poor man came before a judge, and he was crying, and he got a jail sentence. These are not criminals. This can happen to anyone.

I decided that it was my duty as a doctor, as a human being, as a humanist, to offer the help I could. And that decision gave me a great deal of integrity. Suddenly there were women going out of my office happy, relieved, and healthy, and when I compared it to the stories the women told me of the times they went to back-alley butchers—the exploitation, the dirt, the sordidness, the real danger—I had the really good conscience of having helped so many women to protect their lives, their health, their dignity. On the other hand it was very stressful. Because suddenly I was an outlaw.

Now, I knew that eventually this thing would come to court, and I told myself that when it does, I will tell the jury my story, just what I've told you.

MILITANT: The 1973 U.S. Supreme Court decision legalizing abortion had a big effect on your decision to take a public stand, didn't it?

MORGENTALER: Yes, the Supreme Court decision in the United States was historic, so much more than we ever won here. It said that any legislation prohibiting abortion in the first three months of pregnancy was unconstitutional. And that any restrictions in the second trimester could only be justified to protect the woman's health. The highest judicial authority of the United States had recognized the right of women to legal, medical abortion on request.

I wanted to see Canadian women have the same rights as their American sisters. So, I publicly declared in Toronto that I had performed 5,000 abortions without a single death. I made a film of an abortion to educate people that was shown on television. So, I challenged the authorities to prosecute me. I was confident that a jury would acquit me, and this would open the way for safe, legal abortions.

So, in Quebec a French-Canadian, Roman Catholic jury acquitted me [in November 1973]. The jury understood the motivation, they understood the problems of French-Canadian women who could not get a hospital abortion. And they knew of the death and injury women were subjected to. It was a great victory. And I said, well, this is beautiful. The law is going to be blown away.

Well, it's now twelve years later, and we're still battling the same battle.

MILITANT: You were acquitted three times by juries in Quebec before the provincial government relented and declared the law unenforceable, is that right?

MORGENTALER: Yes. The court of appeals of Quebec, in a decision that has no precedent in the annals of British or Canadian jurisprudence, set aside the jury verdict and declared that I was guilty. I was declared not guilty by the jury. But I was then declared *guilty* by the court of appeals. They took away the fundamental democratic right to be tried by one's peers. The Supreme Court of Canada upheld this, and so ten years ago, I went to jail in Montreal for an eighteen-month sentence.

While I was in jail, the government of Quebec decided to bring me to my knees. It wasn't enough for them that I was already in jail. They wanted me to plead guilty. And my lawyer said to me, "Well, Henry, you are already in jail, you have no money to pay me, why don't you plead guilty," and he would raise with the prosecutor that I would get a concurrent sentence. I told him I would never, never, never plead guilty, and he finally understood that he had to defend this as a *cause*, not as a case.

Anyway, I had another trial while I was in jail. The jury came back fifty-five minutes after the judge told them to convict me, and they said, "Not guilty." And here I was after two jury acquittals, and I was still in jail. I remember a cartoon in the newspaper that shows me in a jail cell, with the guard pushing my food under the grill and saying, "Congratulations, doctor, you've been acquitted again."

Well, this created an uproar in Canada, on civil rights. An amendment to the Criminal Code passed that prohibited the court of appeals from nullifying a jury verdict. It is called the Morgentaler amendment, of which I am justly proud. This really extended the civil liberties of Canadians. In particular I remember a union leader in Montreal, with whom I spent lots of time in prison going in and out of court, who had been tried ten times on the same charge. They really wanted him in jail very badly, but juries kept acquitting him. There's no way now for a court of appeals to reverse that acquittal.

MILITANT: And yet you were put on trial a third time.

MORGENTALER: Yes. Because what happened to me violated the new legislation, the minister of justice set aside the guilty verdict of the court of appeals, but ordered a new trial on the first charge! I was already in double jeopardy, here I was in triple jeopardy. I was tried again, and I was acquitted again. And even that wasn't enough. They wanted to try me a fourth time. And I remember very well, people would come up to me and say, "It's terrible what they are doing to you. These are supposed to be representatives of the people." And at the next election [November 15, 1976] the Bourassa government was thrown out and they brought in the Parti Quebecois. [Robert Bourassa headed the Liberal Party, which ran the provincial government of Quebec at that time.]

Anyway, when the PQ government came into power, the new minister of justice declared that henceforth no more trials would be held against doctors for providing safe, medical abortions. Instead the government was going to prosecute the non-doctors who do abortions that endanger women.

And so some of the doctors I trained reopened their abortion clinics, and I opened mine. And then I was approached by the Community Health Centers in Quebec, which provide storefront medicine to people, to train doctors to provide abortions. So now about ten of these institutions are providing abortion services on request in Quebec, under Medicare.

They are in clear violation of the abortion law. My question is: why doesn't the federal government prosecute the government of Quebec for breaking the law, when I am being prosecuted all the time?

By the way, Mr. Bourassa has just been reelected leader of the Liberal Party, and he has started saying that if he is reelected again, he will tighten the screws again, and enforce the federal abortion law in Quebec. Well, he has gotten older, but I don't think he's gotten wiser.

The federal law has to be changed. It is irrational, unfair, discriminatory, and dangerous to women. Why is it dangerous? Because women cannot obtain abortions in many of the provinces of Canada, and when they do, there are usually delays because of the committee system, and the operation comes three, five, eight weeks later than it should. And it's common medical knowledge now that each week of delay increases the danger of complications.

MILITANT: What led to your decision in 1983 to launch the struggle anew, by opening clinics outside of Quebec?

MORGENTALER: In this country, hundreds and thousands of women are not able to get abortions in their own provinces. They come to Quebec Province, to Montreal. Or they have to go to the United States. Recently two women came to my Montreal clinic from Edmonton. That's about 2,000 miles. It costs $800.

And the same happens for the Maritimes. There's one hospital for the whole province of Newfoundland. There's Prince Edward Island, which hasn't got a single hospital performing abortions. The province of Nova Scotia is better, but there is only one hospital performing 90 percent of all abortions. And 27 percent of them are in the second trimester, which is more dangerous. Canada has the second highest percentage of second trimester abortions in the world.

And the situation was getting worse, rather than better. The ability of women to get abortions in hospitals was whittled down by one hospital after another, by pressure from the anti-abortionists, who would organize to get elected to the hospital boards.

The final straw was a lawsuit by one of the leading anti-abortionists, Joseph Borowski, who went to court to try to make all abortions illegal.

So, I thought, instead of fighting him, let's do what we've done in Quebec, where we went ahead and provided services for women that they need. We'll go before a jury, and probably we'll get the same result. And that is the reason why, three years ago, I decided to reopen the campaign by opening clinics in Winnipeg [Manitoba Province] and Toronto [Ontario Province].

MILITANT: You and your associates were brought to trial in Toronto, and in June 1984, the jury came back with a verdict of not guilty, the fourth time a Canadian jury refused to convict you. Did the verdict surprise you at all?

MORGENTALER: Well, I wasn't surprised. I expected it all along. I told them my story from the start, and they didn't take much time to deliberate. It was a tremendous victory for justice, for the women's movement, for the common people. I don't think any jury in Canada would convict doctors in good faith who gave help to people who needed it.

MILITANT: The acquittal in that trial seems to have been a turning point that has put the women's rights movement on the offensive.

MORGENTALER: There's no doubt about it. First of all, we've made a breakthrough in Ontario, which is supposed to be a Tory blue conservative province. The Tories have been in power more than ten years there. Everybody said you couldn't get a jury acquittal in Ontario. But we did win a jury acquittal. The public was very strongly with us. And the big breakthrough is that we reopened the clinic after the acquittal, and we have kept it open. It has been open now for three months, despite the fact that we have been charged again with a criminal offense, despite pickets outside the clinic, and disturbances outside the clinic organized by the Roman Catholic cardinal of Toronto.

And there has been a tremendous movement of solidarity. And hundreds of women have acted as escorts for the patients who go across the picket lines. So all of this has given a tremendous boost to our troops. We know we have the people with us.

We have to fight two main powers: one is the government itself, and the provincial governments. The other is the organized antiabortion movement. They're shrill, they're organized. Their strength is organized mainly in the Catholic Church hierarchy, and in the fundamentalist churches. When I was in Edmonton one day, one of the ministers there said publicly that in order to stop abortions, we could kill one woman as an example to all others! Some of these people are really devoid of humanitarianism, and I really have to fight that.

We have an uphill fight against powerful forces in the government, religious fanatics, antiabortionists, but we all have this tremendous sense of, well, we've finally accomplished something.

MILITANT: There are those who argue that the right-to-life forces are just fringe elements, and the best tactic in dealing with them is to ignore them. Can you comment on that?

MORGENTALER: They can't be ignored, because if you leave them alone, they will take away your rights. You can't let them take away such a fundamental right as a woman's right to abortion. If they take away this right, they might take away other rights as well. You have to stand up to them. And you have to counter their lying propaganda. Otherwise people will accept it. And it's very dangerous. It turns against women, and against people who help them. Basically what underlies all these anti-abortion people is contempt for women, a desire to turn the clock back to the time when women were seen in their stereotype roles as breeders, where women have to procreate year after year, do kitchen work and take care of the children, and nothing else.

I think if we have accomplished anything in our society, it's the legitimacy of the women's rights movement, and the acceptance of the fact that women should be able to be equal partners in society. There is a movement against that. And this movement is reactionary.

And we have to fight that. It's not just a question of fighting for the right to abortion. If women do not have control over their own reproductive functions, they can never develop their other potential. The thing that holds together these antiabortion people—usually they are antiwoman, they are anti-Jew (90 percent of the calls we get that are hostile at the Winnipeg clinic are anti-Semitic), they are anti-Black, they are antiminority, they are antiunion. They are against any progressive forces in society.

And they give themselves this kind of high, moral stance of being "prolife." But it doesn't mean anything: "prolife." What does that mean? Pro-spermatozoa, pro-ova, pro-zygotes, pro-blastocysts, pro-embryos?

They say that every abortion kills a child. This is not true. A blueprint is not a house. This is lying propaganda. So you have to bring the facts of biology to the people, so they understand what's going on. They have to understand that a woman who wants an abortion isn't killing a child. She doesn't want a few cells to *become* a child.

So either we give in and run, or we stand and fight. Either we stop providing services to women who need them, or we take whatever measures are necessary to provide them.

Why Marxists champion abortion rights

BY JOSÉ G. PÉREZ

The following article appeared in the December 20, 1982, issue of
Perspectiva Mundial. It was written in response to a letter from reader P.
Redward, who disagreed with the magazine's support for abortion rights.

P. Redward's letter says that "there are no individual rights that are
above social needs" and therefore *Perspectiva Mundial*'s position in
defense of legal, safe abortion, available to all women, is wrong.

The fact is that the right to abortion—which is simply the
right of women to control their own bodies—is a *very* pressing
social need. That's why tens of thousands of women around the
world have struggled to win this right, and why the Marxist
movement has traditionally backed their demand.

Redward argues the question of "individual rights" and "social needs" abstractly, obscuring the class questions at stake in
the right to abortion.

The issue is not women asserting their "individual" rights
against other "individuals," such as men, or government offi-
cials, doctors, or clergy.

The Hyde Amendment, passed in 1976, cut off federal funding for abortions. This was a major blow against women's rights.

Marxists approach all questions from the standpoint of the interests of the working class. On the question of abortion, we have to begin by recognizing that women are not a group of "individuals," but an oppressed sex. The majority of women in the United States are also exploited as workers.

At the heart of women's oppression is the denial of their right to control their reproductive capacities. That's what the abortion struggle is about—the democratic right of half the population to decide for themselves if and when they will bear children.

Redward ignores the deep-rooted discrimination women face in every facet of their lives.

But only by examining the ways women are oppressed can we understand why this issue is so important, not only for women, but for the working class as a whole.

The majority of women in the United States work outside the home. When they get off the job, they must put in long hours of unpaid overtime taking care of household chores.

On the job, women earn less than two-thirds of what men earn. The yearly median wage of women who work full time is $6,760 less than what men earn. Multiplying this by the forty-five million women in the labor force, we get *$300 billion* that the capitalists make—simply by not paying women as much as men.

For Black women and Latinas, who are triply oppressed as workers, women, and members of oppressed nationalities, the wage disparity is even greater.

Whereas white males have a median weekly salary of $380, Latinas earn only $209.

These differentials go against the interests of the entire working class, because it puts a heavy downward pressure on everyone's wages. Only the bosses profit from this.

In addition, discrimination on the basis of sex—as on the basis of race, nationality, or language—is used to pit working people against each other, placing big obstacles on the road to a united struggle against the exploiters.

Bourgeois ideology justifies discrimination against women on the basis that their "natural" place is the home, performing tasks from rearing children, food preparation and cleaning clothes, to nursing the sick and elderly. This is part of foisting responsibility for all these tasks on individual families rather than making them the collective responsibility of society as a whole. In this way the capitalist rulers and their government free themselves from providing such services as child care, adequate health care, decent education, and so forth.

This is justified by pointing to the biological capacity of women to bear children. Women's main role in society, the capitalists and their ideologists say, is reproduction, while men are the breadwinners, political leaders, and so forth.

What it comes down to is that women must limit their lives to taking care of their children and home, and not become involved in broader society. From an early age, there is a systematic attempt to convince women that they are weak and unintelligent, and therefore should be dependent on men.

There are, of course, physiological differences between men and women. But biology is *not* destiny, as women themselves are proving in the United States and other countries.

Since the rise of the women's movement at the end of the 1960s, thousands of women have entered many jobs they were traditionally excluded from. Women coal miners, truck drivers, steelworkers, and auto workers have given the lie to the claim that these are "men's jobs" only.

In Central America, Nicaraguan women played a key role in the struggle against the Somoza dictatorship. A number of women reached the rank of commander—the highest military rank among the insurgent forces—and played important military leadership roles. In El Salvador, we see a similar process.

Restriction of women's right to control their own bodies is one of the most fundamental and barbaric methods of ensuring that women "stay in their place."

Without the ability to determine whether and when to bear a

child, a woman's entire life is circumscribed by her reproductive capacities. At any time, no matter what her economic circumstances or individual goals, she can be forced to carry a pregnancy to term. Once she gives birth, she will bear the major responsibility for bringing up the child.

Since other forms of contraception are not 100 percent effective, it's no wonder that millions of women choose to have an abortion at some time in their lives.

Without the option of doing this, women's right to full humanity does not exist. Without being able to fully exercise control over their bodies, all other rights—including the woman's right to life itself—are jeopardized.

When abortions were illegal in the United States, rich women could get them from skilled doctors in good hospitals. In capitalist society, there is no law higher than the almighty dollar.

But for most women, the situation was radically different. They were forced to go to back-alley butchers or try dangerous self-induced abortions.

Even following the 1973 U.S. Supreme Court decision striking down antiabortion laws, this right was not equally accessible to all women. This was partly ameliorated by the Medicaid program, which covers some of the medical costs of people on public assistance. But in 1977, Congress's Hyde Amendment went into effect, cutting off Medicaid payments for abortions.

This measure is explicitly directed against the most oppressed layers of the working class, especially women of the oppressed nationalities. It is no coincidence that the first woman to die from an illegal abortion—because she could not afford a legal one following the Medicaid cutoff—was Rosie Jiménez, a twenty-seven-year-old Chicana from Texas.

The Hyde Amendment is part of a broader offensive by the ruling class against the rights and standard of living of working people. Women's right to abortion has been a central target of this offensive.

Redward echoes one idea that has also been raised by right-wing opponents of abortion: "In the *last* analysis, freedom of choice would belong to two persons, since two persons participate in the conception of a new life."

This ignores the fact that it is the woman's body and the woman's life that are most directly and intimately affected by the pregnancy. The man does not carry the fetus within his body; the man will not lose his job or education due to an unplanned and unwanted pregnancy.

Passing a law giving men veto power over a woman's decision to have an abortion opens the door to further state interference. If approval of a man can be required, why not also that of the parents of a pregnant teenager? Or of doctors? Or of a judge?

Redward also argues that "the sexual act is not a question of pleasure. First and foremost it is a natural necessity to ensure survival of the human species."

Human beings are distinguished from animals precisely because we are not slaves of our biology. Scientific advances now make it possible to enjoy sexual activity without fear of an unwanted pregnancy, surely a step forward for humanity.

The logic of Redward's statement would be to adopt the position of the Catholic Church hierarchy that sex without procreation is immoral. This is used not only to oppose the right of women to choose abortion—even to save the woman's life!—but also to oppose all scientific methods of contraception.

The main thrust of Redward's letter is that defending the right of women to control their own bodies means adopting the reactionary standpoint of population-control advocates.

He says, "One billion people could live comfortably in this country; yet there is only one-fourth of that figure, which greatly facilitates the domination of the exploiting minority. As Lenin said: Why not raise sons and daughters so they can fight? Not for nothing has imperialism carried out sterilization campaigns in many underdeveloped countries. The more people there are in this country, the worse will the situation become for the ruling class."

Population-control advocates are often referred to as Malthusians, after Thomas Malthus, a late 18th and early 19th century writer who preached that there was no point in workers struggling for better wages and conditions, since any rise in their standard of living would be automatically canceled out by an increase in population.

History has refuted Malthus so thoroughly that today very few can be found who defend his thesis in its original form. Modern day neo-Malthusians turn his theory upside down in order to arrive at exactly the same political conclusions.

These people say that, while not inevitable, overpopulation is at the root of the poverty of colonial and semicolonial countries and layers of the working class in the United States.

Using this theory as justification, the rulers of the United States have carried out racist "population-control" drives that trample on the right of women to control their own bodies.

Various colonial and semicolonial nations, as well as Blacks, Latinos, and Native Americans in the United States, have been special targets of such campaigns. In Puerto Rico, some 35 percent of the women of child-bearing age had been sterilized by the mid-1970s. Sterilization is so common there that it is referred to simply as *la operación*—the operation. Often women are given incomplete or false information—such as that the operation is reversible—or are made to consent to sterilization as part of the price for obtaining an abortion.

It is easy to show that the neo-Malthusians are charlatans. For example, India is often mentioned as a country that is poor because it is overpopulated, although the real reason is that the British systematically looted it for hundreds of years as a direct colony and continue looting it today in conjunction with the American, Japanese, and other imperialists.

But how overpopulated is India *really*? India has 513 people per square mile. And Britain? 593.

And this is not even one of the more striking examples. Overpopulated Mexico has eighty-nine persons per square mile. Belgium—which nobody ever calls overpopulated—has almost *ten times* as many, with 836 per square mile.

Neo-Malthusianism is an attempt to cover up the fact that behind the poverty of the majority of humanity lies not overpopulation, but capitalist exploitation.

For this reason, Marxists are opponents of neo-Malthusianism. But this does not mean we should adopt a position that would be a mirror image of theirs, calling for maximum population growth instead of zero population growth.

Redward falls into this trap. He argues that population has some decisive relation to the advance of the revolutionary movement. But history shows that what determines whether or not capitalism is overthrown are political factors, above all the degree of organization and consciousness of the working class, and its ability to rally round itself the rest of the oppressed and toiling masses of the cities and the countryside.

This was the point V.I. Lenin—central leader of the October 1917 Russian revolution—was driving at in "The Working Class and Neo-Malthusianism," the article to which Redward refers and which can be found in Lenin's *Collected Works,* Volume 19, pages 235–237.

Lenin describes a 1913 congress of Russian population-control advocates, where one of the speakers exclaimed ironically, "We have to convince mothers to bear children so they can be maimed in educational establishments, so that lots can be drawn for them, so that they can be driven to suicide!"

Lenin explained that this captures perfectly the outlook of the middle classes who, by themselves, can present no coherent program against exploitation and oppression under capitalism. Their call for no more children is both an expression of despair at their situation and an attempt to find an individual way to ameliorate it.

Lenin contrasts this standpoint with that of the workers.

". . . 'Bear children so that they can be maimed' . . . For that alone? Why not that they should *fight* better, more unitedly, consciously, and resolutely than we are fighting against the present-day conditions of life that are maiming and ruining our generation? . . .

"Yes, we workers and the mass of small proprietors lead a life that is filled with unbearable oppression and suffering. Things are harder for our generation than they were for our fathers. But in one respect we are luckier than our fathers. *We have begun to learn and are rapidly learning to fight.* . . . We are fighting better than our fathers did. Our children will fight better than we do, and *they will be victorious.*"

Lenin was not counterposing a different population policy to that of the neo-Malthusians.

And to ensure that there would be no misunderstandings, Lenin added:

"It goes without saying that this does not by any means prevent us from demanding the unconditional annulment of all laws against abortions or against the distribution of medical literature on contraceptive measures. . . . Freedom for medical propaganda and the protection of the elementary democratic rights of citizens, men and women, are one thing. The social theory of neo-Malthusianism is quite another." Lenin championed the fight for women's liberation.

Upon coming to power, the workers and farmers under the leadership of Lenin's Bolsheviks carried out this program and abolished all antiabortion laws. Other revolutionary governments have adopted similar measures. For example, abortion is provided free to any woman who desires one in Cuba.

We believe that in fighting for women's right to control their own bodies—supporting access to abortion and contraception and opposing forced sterilization and reactionary population-control schemes—we stand in the tradition of Lenin and the Bolsheviks.

We believe the struggle against women's oppression is a central strategic question for the revolutionary workers' movement in the United States.

Only by championing the demands of all the oppressed—including defending to the end women's right to control their own bodies—will the U.S. labor movement succeed in mobilizing all the victims of capitalism in a struggle to abolish this outdated social system.

Why the Catholic Church hierarchy opposes women's right to abortion

BY EVELYN REED

The Roman Catholic hierarchy, in the forefront of the antiabortion forces, is enraged by the Supreme Court decision handed down last month [January 22, 1973] that recognizes a woman's right to abortion and rejects the proposition that a fetus is a legal person with rights superior to the mother's.

Immediately after the court ruling, cardinals Cooke of New York and Krol of Philadelphia indicated that they will leave no stone unturned in their efforts to nullify this measure giving women the right to control their own reproductive processes. This attempt to uphold archaic papal doctrine that for centuries has denied women even the smallest measure of control over their own bodies is not confined to Catholics but sweepingly applied to all women under the pretext of the "right to life."

Women should be aware of the basic issues at stake in this challenge. By opposing and seeking to overthrow the Supreme Court decision, the Catholic hierarchy is striving to keep all

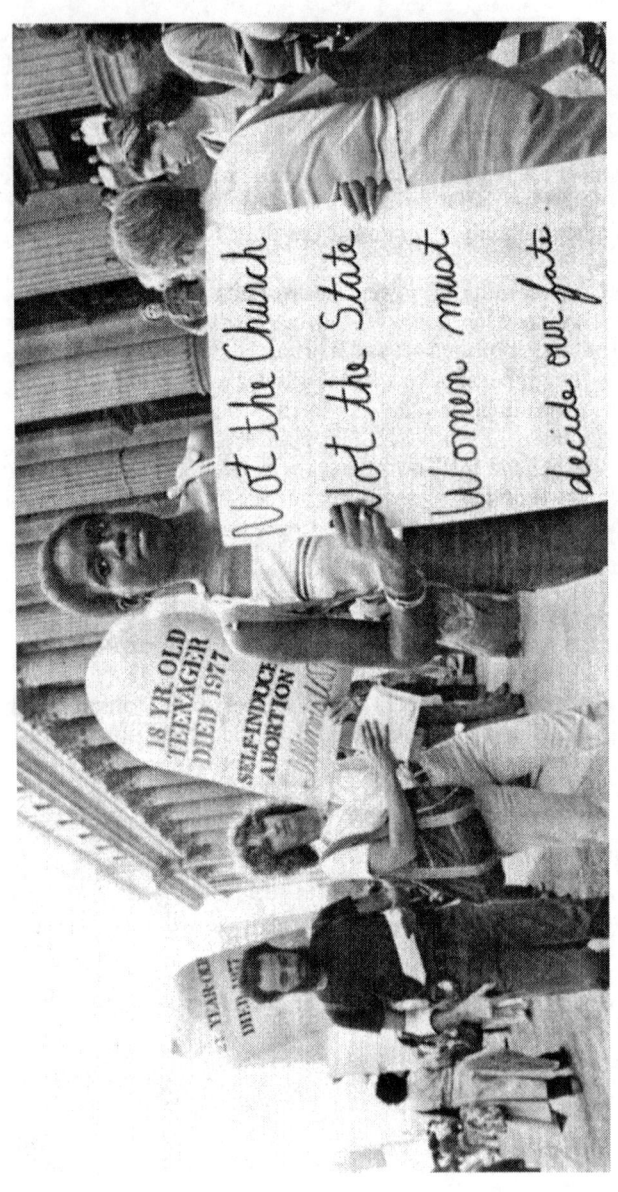

Committee for Abortion Rights and Against Sterilization Abuse (CARASA) picket line in New York City, 1980.

women in the same status as animal females, who are subjected by nature to uncontrolled procreation. They are determined to continue to rob women of their basic human right—the right of control. Let us see why this is so.

All animals are governed by the blind and capricious processes of nature. Humans, on the other hand, alone of all species on earth, can create and control their own conditions of life. Among the other triumphs won over brute nature, humans have learned to regulate their own reproductive processes. The techniques of contraception to limit pregnancies and of birth control through abortion are not to be found among animals. These are exclusively human acquisitions, developed over many millennia of productive and cultural progress. While humanity has grown up out of the higher animal condition, we have long since outgrown our origins.

Animals cannot make tools or engage in systematic labor activities to produce the necessities and comforts of life. By the same token they cannot, like humans, produce new needs along with new techniques nor develop cultural and intellectual standards. Just as animals cannot change raw materials into artificial products to serve their needs, they cannot transform their raw animal nature into human nature and acquire these uniquely human characteristics and aspirations. Animals remain the slaves of nature whereas humans, by deliberately utilizing its materials and processes in productive labor and understanding its laws of operation, have increasingly become the masters of nature.

Among other conquests, humans have broken the chains of animal enslavement to nature's uncontrolled and wasteful mode of reproduction. The most wasteful occurs among the lower forms of natural life. Below the mammalian level, there is little or no maternal care for the eggs that females spawn in tremendous numbers. The ling fish, for example, spawns twenty-eight million eggs in a batch, with only two or three of them surviving in an egg-hungry world to reach maturity.

Mammals are far less wasteful. A lioness usually provides care and protection for her litter until the cubs are old enough to become self-sustaining. The highest form of animal reproduction, closest to the human form, is found among the anthropoids. A female primate bears only one offspring at a time and devotes many months and even years to protecting and raising it.

Despite these differences, *all* animal females, including the higher apes, are subjugated to nature's mode of procreation. They do not have any personal controls or choice in the matter. They are condemned by their biology to proceed from one reproductive cycle to the next, without respite, from the time they reach sexual maturity to the end of their reproductive life when, as a rule, they die. The life of the animal female is restricted to unremitting breeding and little more.

In sharp contrast, the human woman, as a member of the productive and cultural species, possesses the capabilities and potential for acquiring and realizing all the higher aspects and values of human life. Unlike the animal female, a woman need not restrict her life to continual procreation. Modern society now possesses a large body of scientific know-how on birth control that should enable a woman to exercise her conscious, individual choice in the matter. She can decide whether and when to bear children, and how many she will rear. As a human being she can tailor her procreative inclinations to suit her broader needs for a full productive, cultural, intellectual, and political life. Theoretically at least, women have been liberated from the narrow animal existence of continuous breeding.

Unfortunately, while women are no longer the creatures of blind nature, they became the victims of patriarchal class society ever since it came into existence a few thousand years ago. Capitalism remains male-dominated, controlling the lives and destiny of women, benefiting from their exploitation and oppression and, until recently, denying them modern methods of birth control.

While men of the favored classes could assert their rights to a higher human and cultural life, women had to be satisfied with the narrow existence of kitchen, bedroom, and nursery, glorified as the happy home and family. In reality women were degraded to child raisers and domestic servants for men. To keep them in an inferior status, both church and state forbade them to make use of the available methods of birth control. "Keep them barefoot and pregnant" is the most cynical expression of this male supremacy. Heaping insult on injury, women were then told they had been victimized not by class society but by nature, which decreed "biology is woman's destiny."

The struggle of women for control over their own bodies began early in this century and has been pressed forward during every decade up to today. In its first stage the struggle was fought for the partial and limited objective of achieving contraceptive control. Such pioneer feminists in this country as Margaret Sanger, Antoinette Konikow, and others defied imprisonment in their efforts to disseminate methods of limiting pregnancies. Eventually some states legalized contraceptive control devices.

This did not affect the Roman Catholic hierarchy. To the present day papal decrees forbid women of that faith to resort to these methods. Instead they are told to rely on the totally unreliable "rhythm" method. The fact that most Catholic women have caught on to this hoax can be seen by the widespread defiance of the pope's ban. More than two-thirds of married Catholic women practice the prohibited scientific methods, according to a 1970 National Fertility Study.

The second stage of the struggle for women's control over their bodies was very recently opened up by the women's liberation movement. This went beyond contraception control to the demand for the right to abortion. This was not put forward because women prefer abortions to the prevention of pregnancies, but because at the present stage of technical know-how there still exist certain deficiencies in the available methods and devices.

Whether through ignorance of contraceptive methods or through accidental failure of a particular device, women are often trapped in unwanted pregnancies. Under these circumstances the one sure method of birth control is abortion. Should an unplanned pregnancy occur, a completely safe abortion can be performed.

Despite this assured way for women to gain full control over their reproductive processes, legislative, juridical, and clerical decrees against it have prevailed up to the 1970s. Then the key state of New York enacted its liberalized law permitting legal abortions in the first twenty-four weeks of pregnancy. Today, two years later, the U.S. Supreme Court has followed with its ruling covering all fifty states.

Once again the Roman Catholic hierarchy refuses to surrender. It is determined to resist the proabortion movement to the last woman victim of back-alley butchery. The cardinals are fulminating about the millions of unborn who are being denied their "right to life." They hew to the papal doctrine that forbids women *any* measure of control over their bodies and regards the unborn as "sacred" lives, while the lives of the mothers are expendable.

The pope himself made this clear a few months ago when he declared that every pregnancy must be brought to term, even when it is known in advance that a birth will cost a woman her life. This inhuman edict goes far beyond the usual reactionary ban on abortions, which permits the interruption of a pregnancy when a woman's life is endangered. What is behind this manifest hostility toward the female sex by men of the cloth?

They are fearful that if women gain control over their bodies, they will forthwith proceed to fight for full control over their minds and lives. In the course of this struggle, women would shed many of the superstitions, fears, and prejudices indoctrinated into them over centuries of patriarchal rule to keep them on their knees before earthly and super-earthly lords and masters. Even a limited measure of liberation can lead to incalculable consequences—undermining the centuries-old male supremacy over women. This fear of liberated women can be seen in the dire predictions of the cardinals about the "disastrous implications" of the Supreme Court ruling and the "terrifying" developments the decision sets in motion.

This hostility to women is concealed behind the slogan of the "right to life" of the unborn. Such sanctimonious concern covers every germination in a woman's womb no matter how it was implanted—whether through ignorance or by accident, or even by violence on the part of a rapist. Each germination is called a "fetus," and every fetus is called a "person," and every "person's" life is "sacred."

Except the person of the mother. If a mere germination is elevated into a person, the woman herself must be downgraded into a nonperson—a mere receptacle or womb for producing persons. By this criterion, the solicitude for the sacredness of unborn life turns out to be only a cover for reducing a female person, a woman, to the animal level of uncontrolled procreation.

This contempt for women stands out even more clearly when we consider the plight of impoverished and sick women in capitalist society who are economically and physically wrecked by too many births. Nor do the multitudes of unwanted, neglected children fare any better. Robbed of adequate care, protection, and education, what kind of "right to life" do they have? How sacred are the wasted lives of these progeny? Apart from those who happen to be born in well-to-do families, the "sacred unborn" are only *promised* the right to life—a promise that is not delivered. For the essence of *human* life is *not* to be wasted, *not* to be thrust into an animal-like existence.

The black-robed jurists of the capitalist state have made a significant concession in the realm of abortion. The women's liberation movement has won a signal victory with this recognition of women's right to control their own bodies. But the cardinals remain in irreconcilable opposition to the Supreme Court ruling and are mobilizing sentiment to overturn that decision.

We say to them: Stick to your business of controlling immortal souls. But keep your hands off the bodies of women and our democratic right to control our bodies!

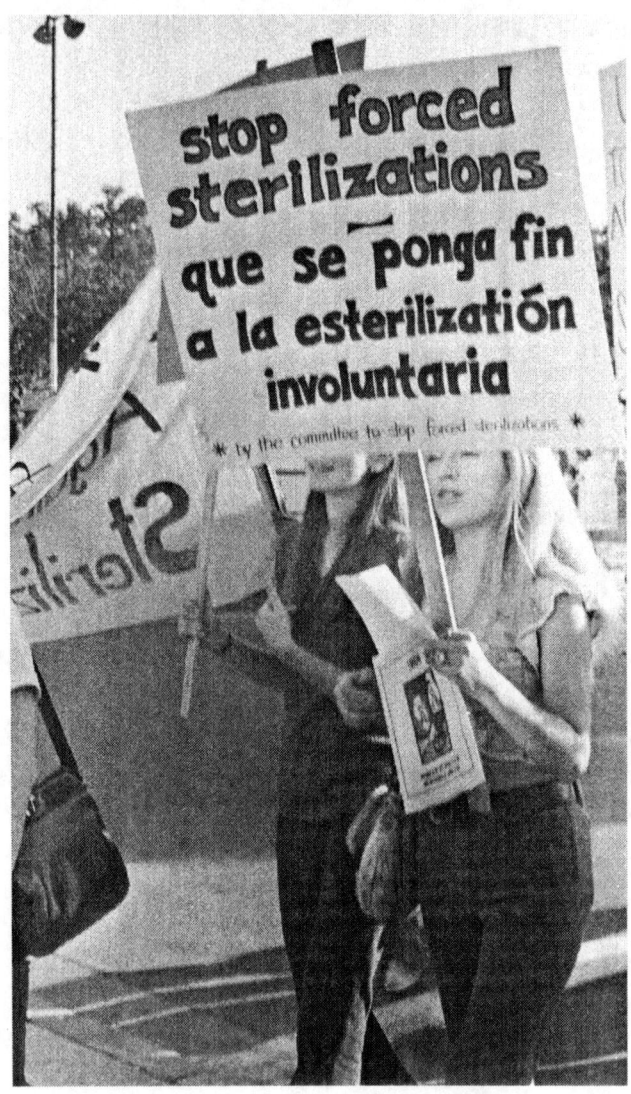

**Demonstration in Los Angeles against forced
sterilization, 1974.**

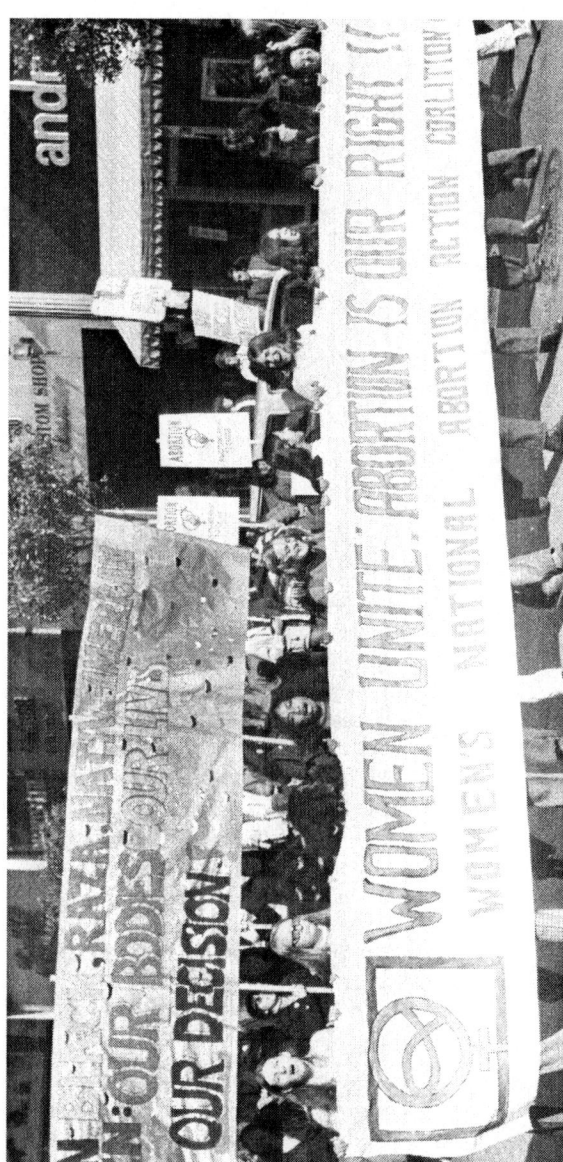

November 1971 in San Francisco. Women's National Abortion Action Coalition (WONAAC) helped lead the fight to legalize abortion in the early 1970s.

from **Pathfinder**

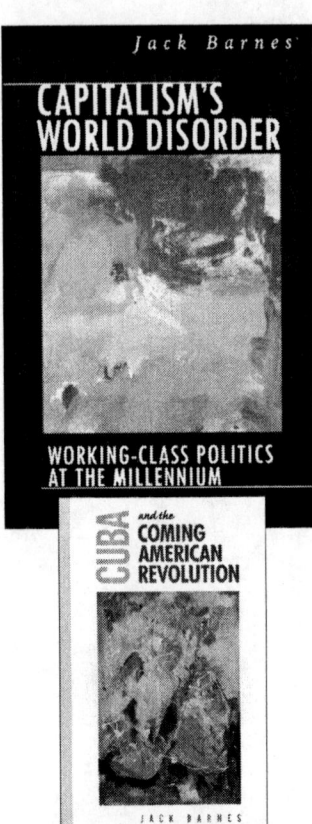

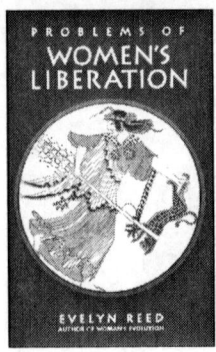

Capitalism's World Disorder
Working-Class Politics at the Millennium
JACK BARNES

The social devastation and financial panic, the coarsening of politics and politics of resentment, the cop brutality and acts of imperialist aggression accelerating around us—all are the product of lawful forces unleashed by capitalism. But the future the propertied classes have in store for us can be changed by the united struggle and selfless action of workers and farmers conscious of their power to transform the world. $24 Also in Spanish and French.

Cuba and the Coming American Revolution
JACK BARNES

"There will be a victorious revolution in the United States before there will be a victorious counterrevolution in Cuba." That statement, made by Fidel Castro in 1961, remains as accurate today as when it was spoken. This is a book about the class struggle in the United States, where the revolutionary capacities of workers and farmers are today as utterly discounted by the ruling powers as were those of the Cuban toilers. And just as wrongly. It is about the example set by the people of Cuba that revolution is not only necessary—it can be made. $13 Also in Spanish and French.

Problems of Women's Liberation
EVELYN REED

Explores the social and economic roots of women's oppression from prehistoric society to modern capitalism and points the road forward to emancipation. $13

The Communist Manifesto

KARL MARX AND FREDERICK ENGELS
Founding document of the modern working-class movement, published in 1848. Explains why communism is derived not from preconceived principles but from facts, from proletarian movements springing from the actual class struggle. $3.95 Also in Spanish.

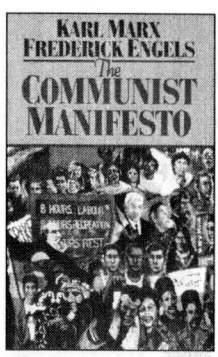

Lenin's Final Fight

Speeches and Writings, 1922–23

V.I. LENIN
In the early 1920s Lenin waged a political battle in the leadership of the Communist Party of the USSR to maintain the course that had enabled the workers and peasants to overthrow the tsarist empire, carry out the first successful socialist revolution, and begin building a world communist movement. The issues posed in Lenin's political fight remain at the heart of world politics today. $19.95 Also in Spanish.

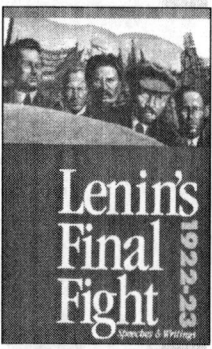

Che Guevara Talks to Young People

The legendary Argentine-born revolutionary challenges youth of Cuba and the world to work and become disciplined. To fearlessly join the front lines of struggles, small and large. To read and to study. To aspire to be revolutionary combatants. To politicize the organizations they are part of and in the process politicize themselves. To become a different kind of human being as they strive together with working people of all lands to transform the world. And, along this line of march, to renew and revel in the spontaneity and joy of being young. $15 Also in Spanish.

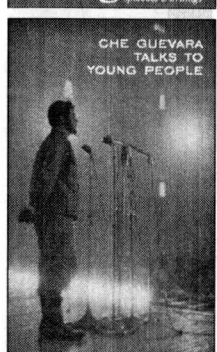

To Speak the Truth

Why Washington's 'Cold War' against Cuba Doesn't End

FIDEL CASTRO AND CHE GUEVARA
In historic speeches before the United Nations and UN bodies, Guevara and Castro address the workers of the world, explaining why the U.S. government so hates the example set by the socialist revolution in Cuba and why Washington's effort to destroy it will fail. $17

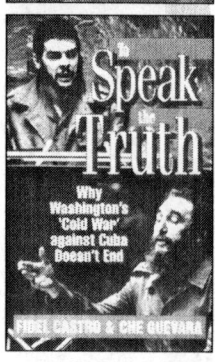

Malcolm X Speaks

Speeches from the last year of Malcolm X's life tracing the evolution of his views on racism, capitalism, socialism, political action, and more. $17.95 Also in Spanish.

U.S. Hands Off the Mideast!

Cuba Speaks Out at the United Nations

FIDEL CASTRO, RICARDO ALARCON

The case against Washington's 1990–91 embargo and war against Iraq, as presented by the Cuban government at the United Nations. $10.95 Also in Spanish.

Art and Revolution

Writings on Literature, Politics, and Culture

LEON TROTSKY

One of the outstanding revolutionary leaders of the 20th century discusses questions of literature, art, and culture in a period of capitalist decline and working-class struggle. In these writings, Trotsky examines the place and aesthetic autonomy of art and artistic expression in the struggle for a new, socialist society. $20.95

The Jewish Question

A Marxist Interpretation

ABRAM LEON

Traces the historical rationalizations of anti-Semitism to the fact that Jews—in the centuries preceding the domination of industrial capitalism—were forced to become a "people-class" of merchants and moneylenders. Leon explains why the propertied rulers incite renewed Jew-hatred today. $17.95

Feminism and the Marxist Movement

MARY-ALICE WATERS

Since the founding of the modern revolutionary workers movement nearly 150 years ago, Marxists have championed the struggle for women's rights and explained the economic roots in class society of women's oppression. $3.50

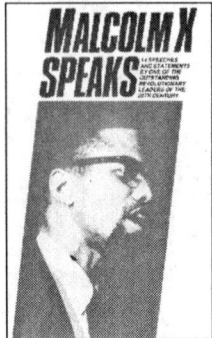 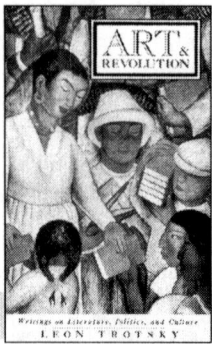 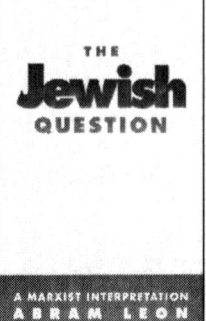